SIZE DOESN'T MATTER AND OTHER WEIGHT LOSS MYTHS

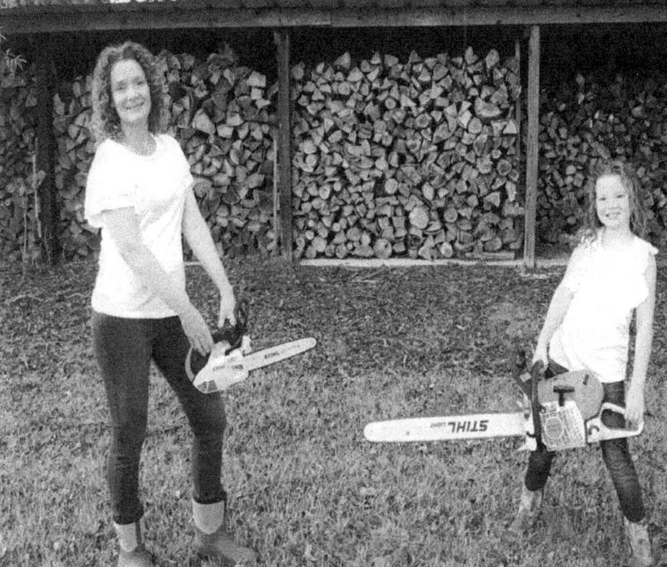

Larry A. Henderson, M.D.

SIZE DOESN'T MATTER:
AND OTHER WEIGHT LOSS MYTHS

ISBN-13: 9781724183231

Published by L Henderson
208 Beaver Creek Rd.
Lucedale, MS 39452
Email: larry@preparingtochange.com
Website: http://mysizedoesmatter.com

Printed by CreateSpace
Available: Amazon, Ingram, Baker & Taylor,
ordinarymiracles.us, preparingtochange.com and bookstores everywhere

Credits
Every attempt has been made to credit the sources of copyrighted material used in this book. If any such acknowledgment has been inadvertently omitted, receipt of such information would be appreciated. Wikipedia is the verification source of all data.

SIZE DOESN'T MATTER: AND OTHER WEIGHT LOSS MYTHS

Larry Henderson, M.D.

A
L Henderson Publication

SIZE DOESN'T MATTER: AND OTHER WEIGHT LOSS MYTHS

Contents

Acknowledgments

Thanks to:

My children, Bailey Renae and Jordan Marie

My wife, Hallie, for showing up in my life, being my best friend, staying by my side, loving me unconditionally, and for having our children

My Daddy, Larry Henderson, Sr., for your never-ending optimism, all of our talks, and all the help that has been so freely given over all my years

My Momma, Elizabeth Ann Henderson, for all the meals, talks, hugs, and taking care of all of us kids and grandkids

My Sister, Leigh Ann Cashwell, for always sticking up for her brother, being a positive role model, and the best sister ever

My Granny, Ina Mae Baygents, for all the meals, walks in the field, rides in the swing, and all the Sundays spent at your house

My Brother-in-law, Matthew Cashwell, for being a great friend, all the spiritual talks, and being a great addition to the family.

Thanks also to Bob C. You'll always have a special place in my heart for your kindness and thoughtfulness.

My nephews, Ori and Luke Cashwell for being great cousins for the girls to play with and wonderful nephews.

Christopher Johnson, III for being my buddy while you were growing up and a kindred spirit.

And last, but not least, Raia King, for being the inspiration and catalyst to make this book happen.

Purpose of this Book

Obesity is at an all-time high in the United States. Seventy percent of the population is overweight. Forty percent of the adult population is obese.   There are thousands of books on weight loss and dieting. Many of these have become best sellers, but the fact remains that these diets don't work for most people. There is so much misinformation out there, that people don't know what to do. Fifty-one percent of American adults want to lose weight. Twenty-five percent are seriously trying to lose weight now (according to a 2013 Gallup survey). I have helped hundreds of patients successfully lose over 10,000 pounds (collectively) using a simple low-calorie diet with an optional exercise plan.   I have seen firsthand what works and what doesn't. I have seen patients fail at weight loss because they believed misinformation they saw on the internet or read in a book. This book will cut through all those myths and get to the heart of the matter. The simple fact is that, if you will follow this diet, you will lose weight. This diet requires no cooking (other than a microwave), no cleaning, is probably healthier than what you are eating now, and costs less than $8 per day total! I have seen it work over and over again. I use it myself when my jeans start getting tight. I try to just eat right and exercise, but I have my weaknesses just like everybody else. When my weight starts to get out of hand, this diet brings it back in line in short order. It has worked for hundreds of people. It will work for you too.

About the Cover – Why Size Matters

Of course, size matters. I had to fiddle with the size of the title font to get it to look right to fit into the space on the cover. My daughter is too small to operate that big chainsaw. The little chainsaw that my wife holds would not work well to cut down a big tree. The big chainsaw would be too heavy to do a lot of overhead trimming. We were shopping for some jeans last night. I picked up some slim fit Levi's, which usually don't fit me. Most of the time it looks like I have been poured into them, but I tried them on anyway. These were a different cut and actually fit which surprised me. My thighs are normally too big. I closed the fitting room door behind me and went to let my wife see me in them. She was on the fence about them but said OK. Her thought process would be a book of its own. Anyhow, I turned around and the fitting room door was locked. I could hear my daughter talking so I banged on the door and started yelling at her to let me in. An alarmed young woman with her son opened the door and explained that my daughter was not in there. Sorry about that. My daughter was behind me talking. I had come out of the next room over. I looked around for an employee to get someone to open the door but didn't see anyone. My daughter saw my predicament and easily slid under the gap at the bottom of the door and let me in. I would have never fit through that space. So yes, size matters. My wife concurs with this, and she says she loves me anyway ☺.

About the Author

I was born in Mobile, AL on April 22, 1974. I grew up in Lucedale, MS with my parents (Larry and Ann Henderson) and my maternal grandparents (Jimmy and Ina Mae Baygents). My paternal grandmother was a nurse and when the doctor that she worked for died, he left me his medical books. I started reading them when I was in elementary school and diagnosed by grandfather with coronary artery disease when I was in 5th grade. He suffered a heart attack shortly thereafter. I knew I wanted to be a doctor from that point forward. I graduated George County High School in 1992. I attended the University of South Alabama for undergraduate, medical school, Family Medicine residency, and stayed on as a teaching physician for a couple years after that. I was there from 1992-2007. During that time, I met my wife. My dad set me up on a blind date after he got an eye exam and liked the optometrist (way to go dad). I came back to work in my hometown when my wife got pregnant with our first daughter (Bailey). Our 2nd daughter, Jordan, was accidentally born at the home because my wife didn't know she was in labor. I'm glad I'm a doctor but would not recommend home deliveries. I am a board-certified family medicine physician with a full-time practice. I have a special interest in weight loss and have helped hundreds of patients in our small town lose weight. I enjoy spending time with family, writing, fixing things, and working on self-improvement. I also enjoy helping other people solve their problems and reach their goals. I am survivor of alcohol and tobacco abuse. I have been smoke free since 2007 and alcohol free since 2015. I maintain a healthy weight (most of the time) even though my genetic report says I am prone to weigh more than average.

I believe that we all have the potential to live life free from bondage. We do not have to be slaves to our appetites. I struggled with smoking until my wife got pregnant with our first daughter. I knew of the effects that smoking had on children because I see it all the time in my clinic. I was not able to quit smoking for myself, but I was able to quit for my children. I quit drinking in 2015 after I had a DUI going to pick up my children from a skating party. I ran out of gas on the way to the party which I can only view as an act of divine intervention since this is the only time I have run out of gas in my car in my entire life. I believe that we are connected with everything around us and that everything we do affects everyone around us. The way we care for ourselves has profound impacts on those closest to us. I can never say, "I'm only hurting myself." There is just no such thing.

There is a spark of divinity inside each and every one of us. May this spark in me, find the spark in you and help you to find the answers you seek.

x

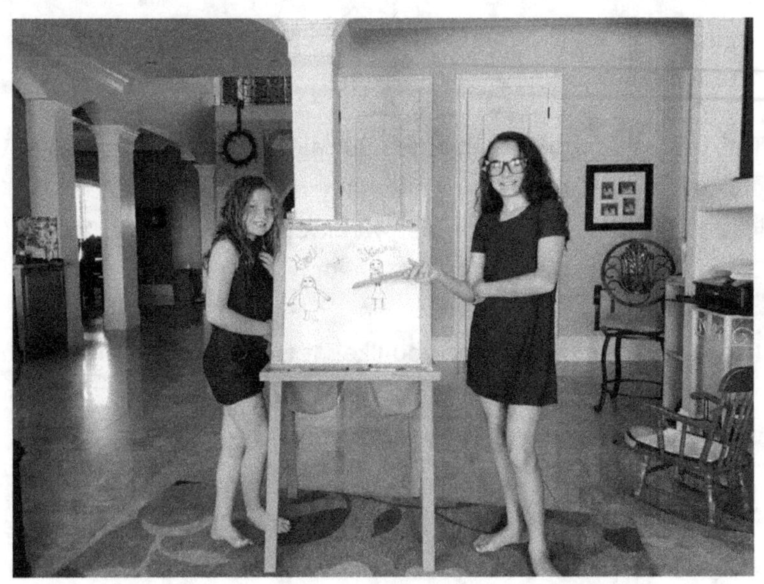

I. The Short and Skinny

The basic framework of the diet is as follows:

Cereal for breakfast (measured; 200 calories)

½ Protein Bar (mid-morning snack; 100 calories)

Frozen meal (Lean Cuisine or others - 300 calories)

Other ½ Protein Bar (mid afternoon snack; 100 calories)

Frozen meal (Healthy Choice or others - 300 calories)

Unlimited Drinks – Water, diet sodas, sugar free tea, black coffee, sugar free flavor packets to add to water, sugar free Kool-Aid

Unlimited Free "Foods" – Celery, broccoli, cauliflower, **sugar free snow cones** (more on this later)

This basic diet provides about 1000 calories per day which is not enough for most people to maintain weight. Many people will lose more than 2 pounds per week on this diet. See the last chapter for your specific calorie needs.

The cereal can be any type you like. It is a good idea to get one that is higher in fiber like Raisin Bran or Frosted Mini Wheats, but Captain Crunch will work (it's just not as healthy.)

Any protein bars are fine if they have about 200 calories.

Frozen meals can be Lean Cuisine, Healthy Choice, Smart Ones, or can be substituted with anything that has about 300 calories. I like these meals because they are easy to prepare, taste good, and get the job done.

You can eat as much of the free foods as you like. I suppose if you ate 10 pounds of broccoli and cauliflower a day, it would mess your diet up, but just snacking on it will not add enough calories to hurt. No added fats or sugars. You can add salt, pepper, and other no calorie spices as you wish.   Sugar free snow cones are wonderful, no-calorie treats. They actually help your body burn calories due to the heat required to melt the ice and bring it up to body temperature. Eating these can actually help you lose weight.

That is the basic starter diet. Go to your grocery store, load up, start eating per the above plans, and watch the weight come off on the scales.

There are some things to watch out for. The main one is low blood sugar in between meals. The protein bars are enough to prevent this from happening in most people. You might find that you need to add another protein bar or granola bar spread throughout the day if you start feeling shaky or like you need to eat. Another caution area is vitamin intake. Most foods are enriched with vitamins in some way, but Vitamin B12 and Vitamin D deficiencies occur in the general population, so you might want to take a daily multivitamin. If you are dieting long term, it wouldn't hurt to see your doctor to get these levels checked. If you have high blood pressure, watch the sodium intake. Try to eat at least fifty grams of protein daily.

Note that a 1000 calorie diet is not enough for most people long term. The tables in the back of the book will show how many calories your body burns daily. The above is just the basic idea that requires very little thought or action to start doing it. The rest of this book will deal with adjusting the diet for your life, give you some ideas, explain why this plan works, and explain how tackling your weight problem can be the first step to a total life transformation.

The words you are reading right now will make neurochemical changes in your brain that will persist forever. Although this book is written in common language, there is a deeper message contained that is transformative in nature. You will never be the same after reading it.

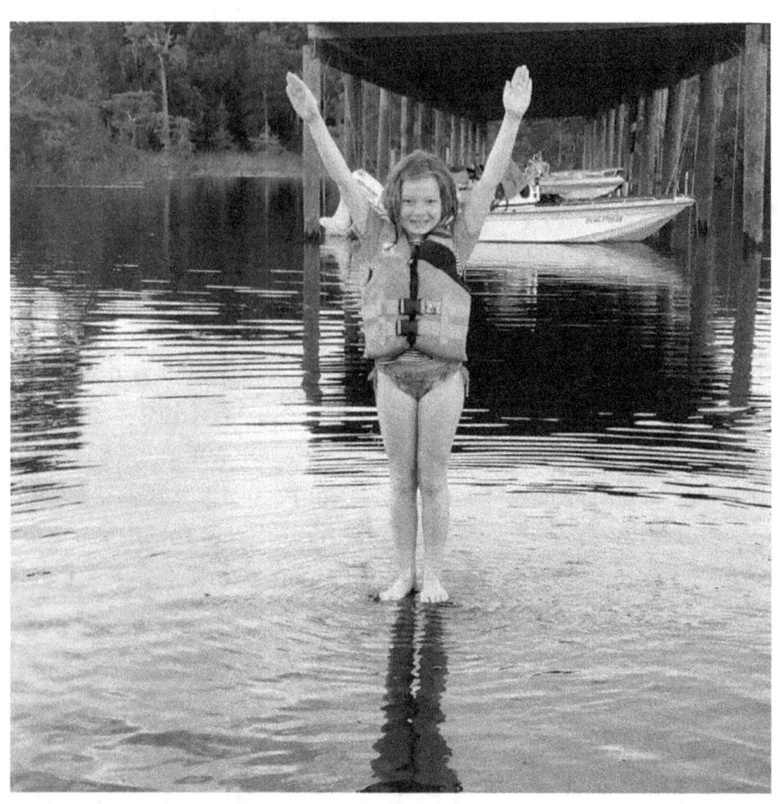

II. Making Your Diet Work for You

This diet works for several reasons. It is easy to follow. **Single serving prepackaged foods** take willpower out of the equation. You eat only what you bring to eat. The decision of what to pack for meals is made beforehand. You don't have to rely on your willpower to hold you back from the buffet or keep you from ordering the big hamburger instead of getting the salad with fat free dressing that you had planned on ordering.

This diet doesn't break the bank. Cereal is cheap. Prepackaged dinners range from about one dollar for Michelina's and Banquet to around three dollars for Healthy Choice, Lean Cuisine, and Smart Ones. You can splurge and get some five-dollar entrees if you are feeling frisky. Protein bars are less than a dollar each. For five dollars a day (total!) you can put together a diet that will get the pounds off. For eight dollars a day, you can have a diet that is tasty, probably healthier than what you are eating now, will have you shedding weight, and wondering, "Why didn't I do this a long time ago?"

Total Calories per day

Flip to the tables in the last chapter of the book right now and look up your total number of calories per day. This will decrease as you lose weight and as you age. Read the instructions, look up your calories, and write that number down below. This is about how many calories on average your body burns daily. This may vary based on your metabolism, but it is a place to start. Figure out how many pounds you want to lose per week. If you want to lose one pound per week then subtract five hundred from your calories burned per day. If you want to lose two pounds per week then subtract one thousand from your calories burned per day. Write these numbers down.

Calories burned per day   ___________

Daily calorie intake to lose one pound per week _________

Daily calorie intake to lose two pounds per week _________

For instance, I am a 44-year-old man, so I flip to the 40-year-old man page. I am 5'9" tall and weigh 170 lbs. I go down to 170 lbs. in the table and then come over to the six-foot column (because 5'9" is closer to six feet than it is to five feet). My calories burned per day is 1800. I would write this on the 1st line. To get my daily calorie intake to lose one pound per week I would subtract five hundred from this which would be as follows: 1800-500=1300. So, 1300 would be my daily calorie intake to lose one pound per week. I would write this number on the 2nd line. To get my daily calorie intake to lose two pounds per week I would subtract one thousand from this which would be as follows: 1800-1000=800. So, 800 would be my daily calorie intake to lose two pounds per week. I would write this number on the 3nd line.

My page would look like this.

Calories burned per day   1800

Daily calorie intake to lose one pound per week   1300

Daily calorie intake to lose two pounds per week   800

I don't have a hard and fast rule for minimum calories, it is better to start at the one pound per week goal and add in a little exercise than to starve yourself trying to lose two pounds per week. Remember, this is a lifestyle change, not a race to see who can lose weight the fastest.

If all you are worried about is losing weight, then calories are all you really need to worry about. Watch the sodium if you have high blood pressure. Choose high protein cereals, meals, and protein bars. The lower your calories, the harder it will be to stick with the diet and get adequate protein. You don't need to obsess over protein. Fifty grams of protein daily is enough for women, and sixty grams is enough for men. Choose a calorie intake that you can live with. I've seen lots of people start off with calories too low. They do lose weight but feel miserable and give up. Whatever you do, do not give up. If you keep your head up and are willing to try something different, you will find your way. **The only way you can fail at anything is to give up!**

You can split the calories up any way you like throughout the day. I like to spread it out over the course of the day because I get shaky (low blood sugar) sometimes if I go too long without eating.

Breakfast

I'm not going to lecture you about breakfast being the most important meal of the day or how breakfast should be your biggest meal or anything like that because I think people just spout that stuff off because they have heard somebody else say it. Who really knows?

What I do know is that breakfast needs to be quick, easy, taste good, and have enough to keep me going until my next meal. For me cereal is the easy answer. I like Raisin Bran and Frosted Mini Wheats. Having fiber in the diet is a good thing for bowel habits, but I eat a variety of cereals. Honey Bunches of Oats, Cheerios, and Kix are OK as well. Less healthy choices might include Captain Crunch and Frosted Flakes due to higher sugar content and less fiber. I use unsweetened soy milk because plant-based products are healthier than animal-based products and it works fine on cereal. Skim milk is fine too. It's best not to use whole milk. Extra fat and sugar are just empty calories and really have no place on a weight loss diet. You will get more than enough fat and sugar in the prepackaged foods, so it is reasonable to cut fat and sugar from the diet where you can.

I could eat a single portion of Kix for instance which would be 1 and 1/4 cups of cereal + 1/2 cup of skim milk which would provide 160 calories. Or I could add another ½ cup of milk to this and end up at 200 calories. Do not pour the bowl overflowing with cereal and fill it up to the rim with milk. This is a common practice, but who knows how many calories you are getting.

If you don't want to measure cereal, you can buy it in prepackaged single serving boxes or bowls (more expensive). If you don't like cereals at all, consider meal replacement shakes like Slim-Fast, protein bars, prepackaged breakfast bowls, or fruits and nuts (but count the calories). Nuts are loaded with calories and fruits are not free foods. Nuts have lots of fat and many fruits have lots of sugar.

Mid-Morning Snack

Eat something in between breakfast and lunch. For me, it is ½ of a protein bar around nine or ten o'clock.   This provides about 100 calories. Any protein bar, or high protein granola bar is fine here. Just find one you like. Save the other ½ of the bar for the mid-afternoon snack. If your calories allow it, you can eat a whole bar for each of your snacks. Drink plenty of fluids. Water is preferred, but if you don't like water, any of the drinks listed are fine. The long-term effects of artificial sweeteners are unknown, so just be warned. We might discover in a couple decades that they are bad for you. Having said that, we know that obesity is bad for you.

Lunch

Prepackaged goodness. Just throw it in the microwave and a few minutes later, you are enjoying a tasty meal. Healthy Choice, Lean Cuisine and Smart Ones all have meals that are tasty, high in protein, low in fat, and not loaded with sodium (salt). The calories on these range from 250 to 400. Just pick something that fits your calorie needs.

If you don't have access to a microwave, you can heat the meal at home and put it into a hot thermos. Consider prepacked tuna (in water) and crackers. Canned soups can be heated and put into a thermos. Just go down the soup aisle and check them out.   Look for higher protein, lower fat, and lower sodium choices.

You can make sandwiches at home. It is pretty easy to figure out the calories in a tuna sandwich if you read nutrition labels. Chips (including baked chips) are available in single serving bags or you can pour some into a zip lock bag.

Red beans and rice are easy to make from precooked rice and canned beans. You can mix these together and microwave for a quick and easy, high fiber, low fat lunch. Canned corn and green beans are great additions. Depending on your calories, you can add a whole can of green beans at lunch or dinner and still be fine. Other canned vegetable like sweet peas and carrots are great too. Just read nutrition labels and watch calories.

Mid Afternoon Snack

The other ½ of the protein bar from the morning or another whole protein bar if calories allow.

Dinner

This is pretty much the same as lunch. Just make sure you eat a variety of foods, so you don't get burned out on one particular food item. You can also cook if you want to. There are tons of skillet meals out there like Hamburger Helper that are easy and taste good. Prepacked frozen vegetables like brussels sprouts, broccoli, and cauliflower can be tossed in the microwave and are a good way to add veggies to the diet. Keeping fruit around the house is a good thing as well. Just watch calories. If you don't know how many calories it has, don't eat it. There are lots of resources that will tell you how many calories different foods have in them. A great resource is **www.calorieking.com**.

Drinks

Water is the best. Drink lots of it. Unsweet tea and black coffee are fine as well.   If you like sweet tea, try Milo's no calorie sweet tea or make your own sweet tea with Splenda. Look at other artificial sweeteners as well like xylitol (available on amazon), NutraSweet, and Stevia. Try them all and find what tastes best to you. There are flavor packets that have very few calories that you can add to water if you want some variety. Again, we don't know the long-term effects of using artificial sweeteners. I use them sparingly.

Free Foods

Celery, broccoli and cauliflower have almost no calories if you eat them plain.   They can be good to munch on if you need something to keep your hands and mind busy. Served raw and chilled, they are crispy and filling. They don't have much taste, but they don't have many calories either.

Sugar Free Snow Cones

These are the ultimate diet food. They taste great. They keep you busy and actually help you burn calories. The secret here is that it takes heat energy to melt the ice. Your body is already expending energy to keep your body temperature at 98.6 degrees. The more ice you eat, the more energy you have to burn to maintain temperature. It requires about 50 calories to bring one pound of ice up to body temperature.   That is one pint of water intake as well. So, eat some sugar free snow cones. For me, the pleasure of eating them outweighs the potential risk of the artificial sweetener. Sugar free Kool-Aid mixed a little strong works well as a snow cone syrup. Or you can make your own snow cone syrup using Splenda and regular Kool-Aid type packets.   Snow cone machines are available on amazon. I have a Hawaiian Ice model that my sister got me for a birthday present when I was in college (best birthday present ever). I think it cost $20 back then and it has made hundreds (maybe thousands) of snow cones over the last 20 years.   The models I saw on Amazon range from $40 (for one similar to the one I have) to $220 for a really nice one.

Note: Eating ice does not cause anemia.   Craving ice can be a symptom of iron deficiency anemia.

Tricks of the Trade

Here are a few pointers to make this journey a little easier for you. They might make it more interesting too.

Spices…. Get some and use them. Salt and pepper can save a bland meal. I don't like bland food. Cayenne pepper, crushed red pepper, and Tiger Sauce are helpful to me too. You'll find your favorites.

Just a few bites and a glass of water. If you are hungry and it is not time to eat, this trick works like magic. Eat a few small bites of something with carbohydrates (crackers, granola bar, biscuit, bread, etc.). Drink 16 ounces of water. Wait 30 minutes. Your hunger will be gone. This sounds crazy, but it is true. This can save you from a serious slip. Just do it. Remember that we make bad decisions when we are hungry, so don't get into a long-term willpower battle with your hunger. It will wear you down. Use this trick to satisfy your hunger in a smart way. I have personally had this work on me. I had eaten very little all day with plans to pig out at a seafood restaurant. I was starving when we got there. They brought out biscuits with honey butter to eat before the meal. I ate ½ of a biscuit and drank some unsweet tea. The place was busy, and they took over 30 minutes to bring our food. By the time the food got there, I was not hungry anymore and couldn't eat much of the meal. Yes, this technique works, even when I don't want it to.

Know your weak points. Don't go grocery shopping when you are hungry. If you can't look at the cookies without buying them, then don't go down that aisle. Be honest with yourself. I can't keep ice cream in the house if there is a Coke in the refrigerator. I have a weakness for Coke floats. I can't make a healthy choice at the cafeteria on a consistent basis if I am hungry when I go there. It's better for me to bring my lunch if I'm trying to eat healthy.

Learn to say "No!" People will offer you food or ask you to go eat with them. If you do choose to eat the food or go out with them, those calories count. It is often easiest to decline the offer. If you do go out to restaurants, order a dish with an appropriate number of calories for your diet. Most restaurants have nutrition information if you ask for it. Realize at the same time that you do not have to explain yourself to anyone. Don't feel like you have to tell everyone you are trying to lose weight. You are not losing the weight for them. Often people will be quick to criticize your failure or constantly remind you that you are dieting. Just follow the diet. Let them come up to you and ask you what you are doing. Imitation is the sincerest form of flattery. If this diet is working for you tell them about it. If it doesn't work for you, keep it a closely guarded secret ☺.

Throw your large clothes away. This is actually very important. As you lose weight and your clothes get looser, you will have to buy some new clothes. Work toward buying smaller clothes. If you keep the larger clothes, it is too easy to slip back into them if you stumble on the diet. While wearing the smaller clothes, if they start to get tight, you know it is time to get more serious about the diet. I will not buy larger jeans. If mine are tight, I cut back on my food intake until they fit again. It works every time.

Whatever It Takes

This diet will not be perfect for you, at first. You will have to modify it to make it your own.   It will show you that it is possible to lose weight.   The calorie tables are based on calculations that represent the average population. You might have a slow metabolism and these numbers might be too high for you. You might have a fast metabolism, or an active job and the numbers will be too low.

You will have to adjust this diet based on your own situation and make it something that will work for you. The bottom line is that there are 3500 calories in a pound of fat (which is what most of us are trying to get rid of). You have to burn 3500 more calories than you consume to burn one pound of fat. You can accomplish this by **eating less and exercising more**. The key to success is not necessarily "working" harder. Form healthy habits and you will just do these things naturally.

Don't give up on the diet.   Don't go back to old behaviors that made you gain weight in the first place. If you are losing weight, but feel weak and miserable on the diet, add some calories. It will slow down the weight loss, but you cannot stick with a diet long term that is making you miserable.

If you are not losing weight after one month of following the diet, then reduce your daily calories by 250. If you are eating less than 1000 calories per day for one month and don't lose weight, go see your doctor for a checkup. Hypothyroidism and fluid retention are possible culprits, but these are relatively uncommon causes of chronic weight gain, especially in younger otherwise healthy people.

The key to losing weight and keeping it off is a **made-up mind** and willingness to do **whatever it takes** to succeed. Let go of your preconceived notions and be willing to try something different if what you are doing is not working.

Exercise

Exercise is not essential for weight loss, but it can help you live a healthier life. I get up about thirty minutes early and do twenty to thirty minutes of exercise six days a week. I have been doing this consistently for over seven years. It has worked well for me. I listen to motivational tapes while lifting weights or watch TV or movies while I am on the elliptical rider.

I don't even think about it anymore. I'm not really focused on the exercise so much. It is just what I am doing while watching TV or listening to some educational audio book. I get interested in what I'm watching or listening to and don't even think about the physical work. I do watch the calorie readout on the elliptical rider just to make sure I am not slacking too much.

I strongly recommend finding a way to exercise on a regular basis for the rest of your life. Twenty to thirty minutes a day really is enough to keep you in shape. Sometimes I stay on the elliptical a little longer if the movie is interesting. I like having the equipment inside my house. That takes away any excuses I might have for not using it.

My routine might not work for you. Find a way to incorporate two to three hours a week of exercise into your routine. It will be one of the best decisions you ever make. You will not regret it. Well, you might regret it if you get run over while riding your bicycle on the highway, your workout partner drops a dumbbell on your head, or if you blow out a knee running marathons. Pick safe, low impact exercises like the elliptical rider, treadmill, light free weights, etc. Don't injure yourself with extreme workouts and you will come to enjoy the way you feel. You'll be able to walk up hills and climb stairs without huffing and puffing. You will be stronger and less likely to get injured.

Long Term Planning

It is not my intent for people to eat TV dinners the rest of their lives, but this diet really works. It is the closest thing to cheating the laws of physics that I have found when it comes to weight loss. It is not the magic answer to living to be old and healthy. I do think it is healthier than the diet that most Americans eat that leads them to obesity.

Here are some resources concerning health and longevity as it relates to diet.

The Blue Zones Solution: Eating and Living Like the World's Healthiest People – Dan Buettner

Eat to Live – Joel Fuhrman, M.D.

www.forksoverknives.com

From reading these books and others, I believe that it is healthier to eat a vegetarian or vegan diet. The above resources show that the more animal products you eat including meats, eggs, and dairy, the more health problems you develop. I do not follow a strict vegetarian or vegan diet, but I do choose smaller meat portions, increase vegetable intake, and

16

use plant-based milk (soy or almond) in place of cow's milk most of the time. I encourage you to do your own research and draw your own conclusions.

Splurge a little!

Face it. We like to eat. We would not have a weight problem if we didn't enjoy eating good food. I like to treat myself some and enjoy eating out with my family from time to time. If my weight is under control, I can indulge myself a little, but as soon as my pants start getting tight, I have to cut back. If I am on the heavy side and trying to lose weight, it is not the time for a treat. It is time to focus and get back to work. I'm not suggesting a yo-yo where you gain and lose weight over and over, but I can enjoy a guilt-free treat when my weight is at or below target.

Mental and Spiritual Health

In addition to taking care of your physical body with diet and exercise, it is important to take care of your mind and spirit as well. If you spend (waste) lots of time playing video games, surfing Facebook, watching mindless television, or videos on the internet, consider trying something a little bit different. Instead of feeding your mind with endless drama and gossip, use your time in front of the screen to do something educational. Listen to an audiobook that teaches you a new skill that might be useful. Self-improvement or motivational tapes can be very helpful. Books on spiritual advancement can be illuminating.

Dare to ask yourself these questions:

Is what I'm doing right now helping or hurting?

Am I doing the best I can?

How can I do better, right now?

What is keeping me from doing better, right now?

Conduct your life in such a way that you can feel good about answering these questions. If I am honest with myself, many times I am not helping the situation and I am not doing the best I can. Much of the time, it is easy to see how I could do better. So, what is keeping me from doing better? When I start asking this question, I must face myself and realize that there is nothing keeping me from doing better right now except my own doubts and fears. Then I can start to do better ☺.

Your life and your dreams are your own. You have a still, small voice within you. It is your true nature and your higher self. It is one with all that is. It seeks peace. Only you can hear or feel this voice. If you are not living your life in alignment with your true nature, it will not let you rest. When you get in alignment with your true nature, you will live your life beautifully and be at peace. This does not mean that you will sit around and do nothing. You will be active. Your actions will be productive and bring results. Only you can know what is right for you. If you try to find your answer by pleasing those around you, you will endlessly chase your tail. Find this inner guidance and follow it. You will **know** that you are doing the right thing.

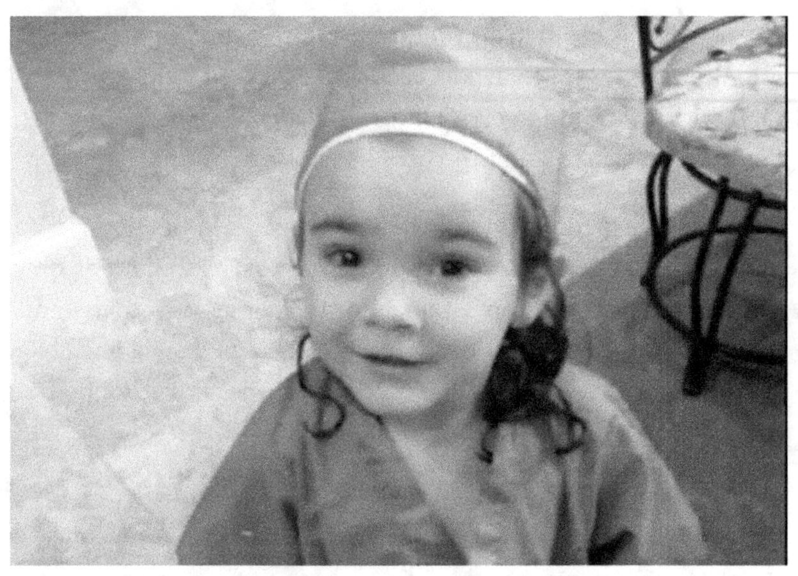

III. Myths – As the Doctor Sees Them

The title of this chapter could just as easily be "Lies – And Why We Believe Them." In my years as a physician I have heard all sorts of stories from patients that are just not true. Are they lying to me? Sometimes yes, but much of the time, I think they believe what they are telling me.   Why would we believe something that is untrue? Very briefly, because we need to. The need to believe a lie arises when we find ourselves in a situation that we have created and need something (or someone) else to blame other than ourselves.

The world we experience is made of three components (physical, mental, and spiritual). The physical part is that which we can see, hear, taste, smell, and feel with our senses.   The mental part is our thinking mind (the voice of our mind) and emotions. The spiritual part is our true self, our inner knowing, and our connection to everything else. It is pure, unconditional love. It is the fabric that the universe is made of.

Most people on earth today live life immersed in the physical and mental realms. They think of the spiritual as something only meant for enlightened masters, ministers, or as something that comes after you die. All of this can get very confusing if we try to figure it out with our minds, and this is where the problem arises.

We are physically just like animals. We have over 95% of our DNA in common with a chimpanzee. We get hungry. We find food. We use the bathroom. We have sex drives. We avoid predators. We seek shelter. All of these are functions of the physical body and the basic parts of the brain. This basic part of the brain contains the reward center that pushes us to satisfy our basic needs for air, water, food, sex, and companionship. We don't need our thinking mind or language to experience and fulfill these basic needs.

Our mental abilities with our large brain set us apart from other animals. We are not only able to experience the things above, but we are able to put them into words and think about them. We can figure out better and easier ways to meet these basic needs. We can come up with better ways to get the apple off the tree. We can even figure out how to grow the apple tree, or better yet, get someone else to do it for us. (It seems dogs have figured out how to get others to take care of them as well.)

The thinking mind opens up a whole new world of possibilities. It is the judging, comparing mind. It not only looks at the external world, but it can look at itself in relation to the rest of the world and compare and judge that too. The problem with the thinking mind is that it must be right. In the animal world, one wrong move can mean death. If an animal fails to satisfy its reward center (air, water, food, sex, companionship), it dies. This fear of death is felt strongly by the thinking mind and is to be avoided at all costs.

The thinking mind sees itself as being above the reward center because it has control of the physical body. The thinking mind has control of your muscles and voice and can delay gratification of the reward center if it thinks it needs to. It appears to be in control of your body. In some ways it is, but in other ways it is not. When we are in extreme danger, or doing something we are naturally good at, the thinking mind is bypassed, and we act instinctively or automatically. This thinking mind can also be thought of as the ego (our sense of identity that views us as being separate from everything and everyone else). It is a component of the physical brain. It works best when we are at peace (well fed, well rested, well hydrated, feeling connected to others, and safe from danger). When we are hungry, thirsty, lonely, tired, afraid, or angry, the thinking mind does not work well. It makes bad decisions to try to satisfy our drives. The reward center is calling for action to satisfy these basic needs and the thinking mind (ego) must come up with a way to satisfy these drives.

If these drives can be satisfied in a healthy manner, there is no problem and we can be at peace. In addition to these basic physical drives, the ego identifies threats, communicates with other minds, and learns from them about what it should and should not do. It learns the rules of society and tries to figure out how to meet these demands as well. It learns, thinks, categorizes, and judges good and evil. It tries to figure out a way to eat and have its cake too.

The mind tries to solve problems. It tries to satisfy all these conflicting drives and demands that are placed on it by the physical body and society. We want to eat good tasting food when we are hungry, but we worry about being fat. Now we even worry about cholesterol, pesticides, sodium, vitamins, and all kinds of stuff. We want to drink, but we worry about fluoride, NutraSweet, and bacteria in the water. We want to breathe but we worry about pollutants in the air. We want to have sex, but we worry about getting pregnant, STD's, and what is acceptable in society. The bottom line is that we want to satisfy the reward center, but we have other things to consider as well. We feel like we have to fit in with the rules of society and please other people.

Foods today are engineered to stimulate the taste buds and be addictive. Companies make them this way. It is hard to eat just a few potato chips or just a little ice cream. The processed sugar and other chemicals short circuit the pleasure center and provide a very strong reward that we want to experience over and over again. This is similar to how drugs and alcohol stimulate the reward center. This good feeling blots out all our negative feelings for a short period of time and we want to feel it over and over again. This can get out of hand. People can continue to eat food to make themselves feel good to the point that they become overweight and start to have health and image problems. The same goes for drugs and alcohol. If used in moderation, everything is fine, but when drugs and alcohol become the focus of life, alcoholics and drug addicts are born. There are great parallels between food addiction and drug/alcohol addiction. If you are having consequences because of overeating (diabetes, obesity, high cholesterol, knee or foot problems, feeling like you have a problem with eating, or poor self-image) and you have tried to control or cut down on your food intake without success, then you suffer from food addiction (which is a spiritual problem). If this is the case, I have written another book called **Preparing to Change** that deals with addictions (including food addiction) which is beyond the scope of this book.

The following is a modification of the CAGE questionnaire which is used to identify people that have a problem with drinking. I have just changed alcohol to food (which would include drinks with calories like sweet tea, milkshakes, milk, and soft drinks.)

Have you ever felt you should cut down on your eating (or calorie containing drinks)?

Have people annoyed you by criticizing your eating habits?

Have you ever felt bad or guilty about your eating?

Have you eaten to relieve stress or because you were "bored?"

Scoring: You score 1 point for every yes answer to the above questions. A score of 2 or greater is clinically significant with higher numbers being associated with a problem with food.

When I answer these questions, my score is 3. I have been overweight and felt like I needed to cut down on my eating. I can't recall being criticized (at least not to my face) about my eating habits. I have felt guilty about eating a Coke float when I was trying to diet. I have definitely eaten to relieve boredom. Addiction to food can be defined as having limited control over your intake of food, having a desire to cut down on food intake, and having negative consequences at a result of overeating (i.e. being overweight or obese, poor self-image, health problems, etc.) With fifty-one percent of adult Americans wanting to weigh less than they do now, American has a problem with food addiction, just like we do with alcohol, tobacco, and drugs.

With all that being said, here are some of the myths I have heard in my weight loss clinic over the years and a response that debunks it.

Myth: I don't eat that much.

What It Implies: It is not my eating that is causing me to be overweight. It must be something else. It might be my metabolism or my hormones. I am overweight for some mysterious reason that just can't be explained.

My response: Yes. You do eat that much. You have consumed more calories than your body burns for an extended period and those excess calories have been stored as fat. Calorie intake is the sole cause of weight gain.

Test: Get up one morning. Weigh yourself. Do not consume any calories at all. Drink only water. This is called a water only fast. Do this for three days and see what your weight does. Then start eating and see what your weight does. Check with your doctor before you do this to make sure it is safe. There is no need to do this test. You know that if you don't eat you will lose weight. But if you do decide to try this out and you gain weight on the water only diet, come see me.

Myth: You have to eat in order to lose weight.

What It Implies: If I don't eat my metabolism will slow down and I will gain weight. I need to eat to keep my metabolism up. That way I can lose weight.

My response: You do not have to eat to lose weight. When you are eating is the only time you are gaining weight. I believe it is true that eating frequent small meals will help boost metabolism and is healthier than eating one large meal a day. I have personally witnessed that when people get sick and are unable to eat, they lose weight. Sometimes it is so bad we must feed them with tubes to prevent them from losing weight. Look at countries where people don't have enough to eat. They are all skinny. Not eating does not slow down metabolism that much.

Test: Go out and eat a lot of food for a week. Eat multiple large meals daily (five or more). Supplement with frequent snacks and protein shakes. See what your weight does. If you lose weight on this plan, come see me.

Myth: I am in a bad position. I can't exercise due to my bad knees. So, there is no way I can lose weight.

What It Implies: Exercise is essential to lose weight. I might as well give up. I wish I could, but it is totally out of my hands. Poor, poor me. There is nothing I can do. Oh well.

Reality: Exercise is not essential to lose weight. I think exercise is a good idea. I exercise 6 days per week (20 minutes per day). The calorie tables in this book are for people that do not exercise. They show how many calories you burn if you don't even get out of bed in the morning. If you lay in bed around the clock, your body burns calories just to keep your heart pumping, kidneys filtering, lungs breathing, and your brain thinking. Even if you have bad knees, you could do exercise with your arms.

Test: Follow a low-calorie diet as suggested in the first two chapters for one month. If you are not losing weight, then decrease your daily caloric intake by 250 per day. Do this for three months and see where your weight goes.

Myth: Prepackaged foods are not healthy. They are too high in sodium and will raise my blood pressure. I can't eat just that.

What It Implies: I can't follow a diet like this. It is too dangerous. I better stick with what I'm doing (never mind the fact that it is not working).

My response: It is true that prepackaged foods are often high in sodium and you do need to watch labels. Monitor your blood pressure. Most people will tolerate sodium intakes near the maximum recommended daily allowance without problems. Again, if you have high blood pressure, choose lower sodium products (which are available). Prepackaged food options are a lot healthier than they were twenty years ago.

Test: Just try the diet out and see what your blood pressure does as you lose weight. Watch your cholesterol numbers improve as well.

Myth: I can't lose weight. I've tried everything.

What It Implies: I have tried every method that has ever been created to lose weight and none of them worked.

My response: You have not tried everything. I know you have not tried this diet, or you would have lost weight. It is impossible to gain weight if you are eating less calories than your body burns over the long term.

Test: Follow this diet for three months, cutting calories as described if you fail to lose weight after the first month.

Myth: My obesity is not causing me any problems.

What It Implies: The rules do not apply to me. I can remain overweight with no consequences.

My response: If you are truly fine with your weight, then you do not have a self-image problem (which is wonderful). I would still challenge you to look at some objective research on obesity and see if you might be at increased risks of health issues down the road (even if you are currently not having problems). Remember smoking, alcohol, drug use, gambling, and overspending don't cause problems immediately, either.

Test: Look on the internet at all the disorders that obesity increases your risk of having. Do you have any of these problems?

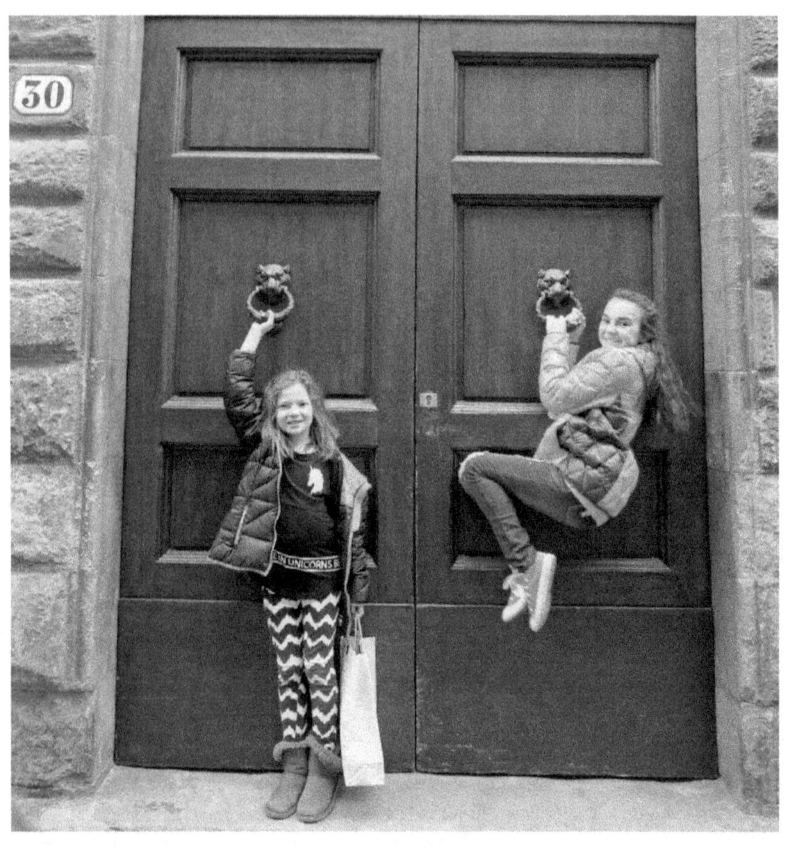

IV. Modern Barriers to Success

Too much information

There is too much conflicting information out there. One diet says this, another says the exact opposite. Some studies show eating nuts (which are loaded with calories) will not cause weight gain. Some studies show low carb is the way to go. Some show low fat.   Different people are quick to give advice. They have all kinds of patches and supplements. Any of these will work if they include a plan that causes you to eat less and exercise more. You must burn more calories than you take in. The supplements you take do not change this basic fact. Are you really going to take advice on how to lose weight and keep it off from a person that is overweight? If you want to take advice from someone, find someone that was obese and solved their problem in a way that you would like to solve it. What works for one often works for another. The key is **believing that you can lose weight**.

Long books

Why do you need a 200-page book to tell you to eat less and exercise more? If people were motivated enough to read a book that long and follow the instructions, they would have solved their weight problem long ago. Now, if you listen to the book on audio while you are riding an elliptical rider, you might be on to something.

Quick Fixes

We live in a world of instant gratification and want results without having to do the work. This book is an attempt to give you a realistic quick fix, because none of the fad diets really deliver on the ridiculous claims that they make. I had one patient lose over fifty pounds in two months. It was an amazing transformation. I saw it with my own eyes. He went from over 300 pounds down to 245 pounds by exercising and going on a low-calorie diet. His results are not typical. I don't expect everyone else to have these results, but I do see motivated patients lose twenty pounds in two months quite frequently.

This is done mostly with cutting calories and exercise sprinkled in, but some do it with no exercise.

People like the idea of weight loss surgeries and diet pills. These are less desirable solutions. The surgeries have permanent side effects like only being able to eat a few bites at the time, vitamin deficiencies, and rarely infection and death. Diet pills are just a band-aid. They can be good to help someone get started and get some motivation, but many people use them as a quick fix and then gain the weight back when they get off the medication. This is not a healthy long-term solution. Think of this as a lifestyle change rather than a diet. Use this as a starting point and modify it to work for you. You can make it healthier as time goes on.

Nay-sayers (Do it anyway)

People in your life will try to console you and comfort you and make you feel better about your weight problem. They will point out that it is not your fault and that you are not *too* overweight. You can look around and find people heavier than you and deny that you have a problem. If you don't have a problem, there is no need to act.

Others will tell you that it is genetic, and you are just destined to be overweight. They will tell you that you will fail. Even some of your closest loved ones will not believe in you.

Anytime you are trying to improve yourself or do something great, there will be nay-sayers. When I was writing this book, I was shocked to have one whom I love dearly and is always so supportive and optimistic about everything tell me to not quit my day job. When asked what he meant by this, the response was that I would not succeed in meeting my goals with this book. So, I wrote it anyway.

You absolutely can do it. There is a power inside you that is greater than you can imagine. May this book awaken that power and find you on your way to accomplishing your goals.

Friends, Family, and Food Joints

In the United States, we eat at many social occasions. It is always somebody's birthday, or some get together that involves eating. They bring lunch to our office frequently. It is usually very good tasting, but rarely healthy. Cafeterias and restaurants may offer healthy solutions, but it is difficult to make a healthy choice when we are hungry. All of these are situations to avoid if you are trying to lose weight. Remember that when you are hungry or excited, your brain will not make good decisions and you might find yourself eating things that you later regret.

I'll just have one……I'll start my diet tomorrow….I'll start exercising tomorrow

Sounds good, but you won't do it. Do better today. I can't tell you how many times I have intended to do something better tomorrow, only to fail and put it off another day and another…. **Do it today. All you have is today.** It doesn't matter what you did yesterday, and you don't know what tomorrow will bring. Do better today and leave yourself in a better position tomorrow. Habits are formed one action and one day at a time. Are your actions today forming habits that will benefit you in the days to come or are you indulging today and creating consequences that you will have to deal with tomorrow? Do yourself a favor and **do better today**.

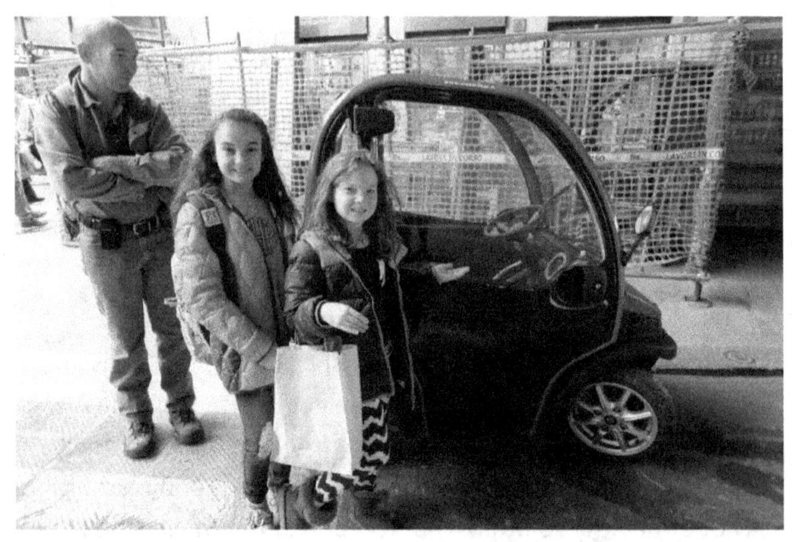

V. Why Size Really Matters and Some Ways It Shouldn't

Some Ways That Size Shouldn't Matter

I read an article online at diversitywoman.com that said discrimination against plus-sized individuals is as common as racial discrimination. Women who are classified as obese generally earn less than thin women. They are also less likely to be hired. A 2005 survey of human resource personnel in the UK reported that 93 percent said they would choose a thin applicant over a plus-size one "purely on the basis of their weight." It also talked about how devastating it can be for someone to be lectured about their weight just because someone else does not like the way that they look because they are overweight.

I do not support discrimination of any kind. I remember seeing obese kids get picked on when I was in school. These personal attacks are totally unwarranted. People that engage in the behavior of putting other people down to make themselves feel better are insecure themselves. They do not feel good about themselves, so they must find ways that others are inferior to them. This gives them some pathetic justification that they are superior. A person's size does not in any way lessen their value as a human being. We are all part of the same whole. We are all in the same boat, trying to do the best that we can with the cards that life has dealt us. It is in everyone's best interest that we support and love each other and remember that we are all one. When I make fun of or hurt another person, I am hurting myself.

Some obese people are perfectly content to be that way.   They are not aware of any health problems related to obesity and have no desire to change their behavior. They do not have a problem with their self-image.

Some people with a normal body weight think that they are too fat or too thin. They do have a problem with weight based on their self-image.   Unfortunately for these folks, adjusting weight rarely fixes their "weight" problem, because their "weight" problem has been incorrectly identified as a weight problem when it is really a self-image problem.

Some people who are underweight think they are overweight. They use dangerous diets, laxatives, and vomiting to induce weight loss. This type of self-image problem leads to all kinds of physical problems. Again, changes in weight will not fix this problem as it is a self-image problem.

Why Size Really Matters

Obesity is defined as Body Mass Index >30. Overweight is defined as Body Mass Index >25.

People with obesity compared to those with a healthy or normal weight, are at increased risk for many serious diseases and health conditions including the following;

- All causes of death (mortality)
- High blood pressure (hypertension)
- High LDL (bad cholesterol), low HDL (good cholesterol)
- Type 2 Diabetes
- Coronary heart disease
- Stroke
- Gallbladder disease
- Osteoarthritis (breakdown of cartilage in joints)
- Sleep apnea and breathing problems
- Some cancers (endometrial, breast, colon, kidney, gallbladder and liver)
- Low quality of life
- Mental Illness (depression and anxiety)
- Body pain and difficulty with physical functioning

Nearly 9 out of 10 newly diagnosed Type 2 diabetics are obese.

Obesity also has significant economic impacts. In 2008 dollars, the annual costs of medical care for obesity was estimated at $147 billion. The annual cost of obesity-related absenteeism from work ranges from $3.38 billion to $6.38 billion.

The above information is abstracted from CDC.gov.

This data shows that obesity is harmful to the individual and society as a whole. In addition to these facts supported by hard data, there are other adverse effects of obesity on the individual and those around them. I cannot stress enough, that I am not writing this to judge anyone, just to educate. Since obesity means higher risk of debilitating health problems including heart attacks, diabetes and strokes, this means that family members of obese individuals have to devote more time and resources to aid in the care of that person. I see this every day in my office. I see morbidly obese patients being pushed into the office by their sons, daughters, spouses, siblings, or parents. Concerned family members devote their precious time and energy to helping care for health problems related to obesity. They might know that obesity is contributing to these problems but are hesitant to say anything for fear of hurting their loved one's feelings.

Family members often worsen the problem by continuing to bring unhealthy food to the obese person. In recovery circles, this is called "enabling." Bizarre family dynamics occur. Family members cater to the obese individual, which only makes the problem worse. I had one patient that was so far gone that he never got out of his chair even to take a bath. People brought him food. He gained to over five hundred pounds. He only came to the doctor when he suffered a blood clot in his leg that went to his lungs and he became severely short of breath. I have often wondered what he would have done if someone would have quit bringing him too much food and perhaps brought him a diet closer to what is outlined in this book to help him lose weight.

There is a strong belief that "This is my body. I am only hurting myself." As a recovering alcoholic, I have had to face this lie directly. When the effects of my alcohol abuse on my family were staring me in the face and I could no longer fool myself that my drinking was not hurting anyone else, I knew I had to change. I became willing to do **whatever it took** to stop drinking, **no matter what**. For me this meant inpatient rehab. In retrospect, this was the best thing that ever happened to me.

Gallup conducts an annual Health and Healthcare survey. In 2013 it showed that 51% of adult Americans want to lose weight, but only 25% were seriously trying to lose weight. This data shows that MOST adult Americans want to lose weight. This is not just 51% of overweight or obese people. This is 51% of the people surveyed.

From this data, it is safe to say that these people that want to lose weight have a reason for wanting to lose weight. It could be to improve their health, reduce knee pain, improve self-image, fit into some smaller jeans, or to be able to fit into a regular sized chair. They might want to lose weight due to pressure from family members or because their doctor told them to. Whatever the reason, it is not enough of a motivator to make people seriously try to lose weight. There could be several reasons for this. The most likely reason in my mind is that people perceive that it is too much work or that they just can't do it. Many people have tried to lose weight, only to gain it back. Many have wasted money on supplements or tried to follow fad diets and failed. For whatever reason, they have given up.

If you are reading this book, I assume that you have not given up. That means you can do it. If you will follow the diet outlined in this book, you can safely lose weight while still getting to eat food that tastes good and have some treats along the way. Most of the hard work is done on the front end when you go spend thirty minutes at the grocery store each week picking up foods you like to eat.

Quit chasing your tail (author unknown)

The wise old cat walked up on a kitten that has chasing his tail. Round and round he went.

The old cat asked, "Why do you constantly chase your tail?"

The kitten replied, "I learned in school that happiness is in the end of my tail. If I can catch it and hold on to it, I will be happy."

The wise old cat replied, "I learned too that happiness is in the end of my tail, and that whenever I am doing what I am supposed to be doing, it follows me everywhere I go."

Quit chasing your tail and start doing what you are supposed to be doing and let happiness follow everywhere you go.

Body Mass Index Table

The table on the following page is a table that will show your Body Mass Index (BMI). Twenty-five and over is considered overweight. Thirty and over is obese. Simply look at your weight in pounds and height in inches. The shaded area shows Body Mass Index greater than or equal to twenty-five.   If your BMI falls in the shaded area, you could benefit from losing weight. The lower limit of a healthy BMI is 18.5.

It is interesting that the healthy range is 18.5-24.9 for both men and women. My wife and I are both about 5'9". I weight 170 lbs. and she weighs 145 lbs. I am at the upper limit of a healthy normal weight and she is closer to the middle. If I lost down to 145 lbs., I would probably look too thin and if she gained to 170 lbs., she would probably look overweight. This is just a perception and may just be an example of how our idea of what is "normal" gets formed by what we are exposed to in our daily lives.

I personally think there does need to be adjustment based on gender because men generally have more muscle mass and women have a higher percentage of body fat, but this is just my opinion. From a medical standpoint a BMI from 18.5-24.9 is considered healthy, so just use your own judgement as to where you would like to be in this range.

Weight	Height (inches)												
	56	58	60	62	64	66	68	70	72	74	76	78	80
110	25	23	21	20	19	18	17	16	15	14	13	13	12
120	27	25	23	22	21	19	18	17	16	15	15	14	13
130	29	27	25	24	22	21	20	19	18	17	16	15	14
140	31	29	27	26	24	23	21	20	19	18	17	16	15
150	34	31	29	27	26	24	23	22	20	19	18	17	16
160	36	33	31	29	27	26	24	23	22	21	19	18	18
170	38	36	33	31	29	27	26	24	23	22	21	20	19
180	40	38	35	33	31	29	27	26	24	23	22	21	20
190	43	40	37	35	33	31	29	27	26	24	23	22	21
200	45	42	39	37	34	32	30	29	27	26	24	23	22
210	47	44	41	38	36	34	32	30	28	27	26	24	23
220	49	46	43	40	38	36	33	32	30	28	27	25	24
230	52	48	45	42	39	37	35	33	31	30	28	27	25
240	54	50	47	44	41	39	36	34	33	31	29	28	26
250	56	52	49	46	43	40	38	36	34	32	30	29	27
260	58	54	51	48	45	42	40	37	35	33	32	30	29
270	61	56	53	49	46	44	41	39	37	35	33	31	30
280	63	59	55	51	48	45	43	40	38	36	34	32	31
290	65	61	57	53	50	47	44	42	39	37	35	34	32
300	67	63	59	55	51	48	46	43	41	39	37	35	33
310	69	65	61	57	53	50	47	44	42	40	38	36	34
320	72	67	62	59	55	52	49	46	43	41	39	37	35
330	74	69	64	60	57	53	50	47	45	42	40	38	36
340	76	71	66	62	58	55	52	49	46	44	41	39	37
350	78	73	68	64	60	56	53	50	47	45	43	40	38
360	81	75	70	66	62	58	55	52	49	46	44	42	40

Calories Burned Per Day Tables

The table on the following pages will help you estimate your calories burned per day. These numbers are based on the Harris-Benedict Equation. There are lots of energy expenditure equations out there. If you want to use a different one, you can find them online and use them for this diet. The numbers on these tables are just the plain basal metabolic rate. They do not consider ANY activity. This is an estimate of calories burned if you simply stayed in bed around the clock and ate. If you move around ANY, you are burning more calories than these tables show. This is just a starting point. You will probably need to add more calories as you get into the diet. It is better to underestimate calories. When you see weight come off the scales, it will give you motivation. You can increase calories as needed. Just go to the page that is closest to your age. Note the gender in the upper right-hand corner. Go over to the column that is closest to your height (i.e. 5'5" would be 5 feet and 5'7" would be 6 feet). Then go down to the row that is across from your weight in pounds. This is your Calories Burned per Day that you will put on the line in Chapter 2. This is only a starting point. It will generally be an underestimate of how many calories you burn, but if your Calories Burned per Day is greater than 2500, just use 2500 for your Calories Burned per Day. If you exercise, you can figure out how many calories you are burning with exercise and add that to your Calories Burned per Day. I burn less than 500 calories daily with formal exercise, so I just ignore calories burned by exercise. If I start losing too much weight, I just eat more (this is not a problem).

Weight (lbs)	20 year old Man			
	Height (feet)			
	4	5	6	7
110	1200	1400	1500	1700
120	1300	1400	1600	1700
130	1300	1500	1600	1800
140	1400	1600	1700	1900
150	1500	1600	1800	1900
160	1500	1700	1800	2000
170	1600	1700	1900	2000
180	1700	1800	2000	2100
190	1700	1900	2000	2200
200	1800	1900	2100	2200
210	1800	2000	2100	2300
220	1900	2100	2200	2400
230	2000	2100	2300	2400
240	2000	2200	2300	2500
250	2100	2200	2400	2500
260	2100	2300	2500	2600
270	2200	2400	2500	2700
280	2300	2400	2600	2700
290	2300	2500	2600	2800
300	2400	2600	2700	2900
310	2500	2600	2800	2900
320	2500	2700	2800	3000
330	2600	2700	2900	3000
340	2600	2800	3000	3100
350	2700	2900	3000	3200
360	2800	2900	3100	3200

	30 year old	Man		
	Height (feet)			
	4	5	6	7
Weight (lbs)				
110	1200	1300	1500	1600
120	1200	1400	1500	1700
130	1300	1400	1600	1700
140	1400	1500	1700	1800
150	1400	1600	1700	1900
160	1500	1600	1800	1900
170	1500	1700	1800	2000
180	1600	1800	1900	2100
190	1700	1800	2000	2100
200	1700	1900	2000	2200
210	1800	1900	2100	2200
220	1900	2000	2200	2300
230	1900	2100	2200	2400
240	2000	2100	2300	2400
250	2000	2200	2300	2500
260	2100	2300	2400	2600
270	2200	2300	2500	2600
280	2200	2400	2500	2700
290	2300	2400	2600	2700
300	2400	2500	2700	2800
310	2400	2600	2700	2900
320	2500	2600	2800	2900
330	2500	2700	2800	3000
340	2600	2800	2900	3100
350	2700	2800	3000	3100
360	2700	2900	3000	3200

Weight (lbs)	4	5	6	7
		40 year old Man		
		Height (feet)		
110	1100	1300	1400	1600
120	1200	1300	1500	1600
130	1200	1400	1500	1700
140	1300	1500	1600	1800
150	1400	1500	1700	1800
160	1400	1600	1700	1900
170	1500	1600	1800	2000
180	1600	1700	1900	2000
190	1600	1800	1900	2100
200	1700	1800	2000	2100
210	1700	1900	2000	2200
220	1800	2000	2100	2300
230	1900	2000	2200	2300
240	1900	2100	2200	2400
250	2000	2100	2300	2400
260	2100	2200	2400	2500
270	2100	2300	2400	2600
280	2200	2300	2500	2600
290	2200	2400	2500	2700
300	2300	2500	2600	2800
310	2400	2500	2700	2800
320	2400	2600	2700	2900
330	2500	2600	2800	2900
340	2600	2700	2900	3000
350	2600	2800	2900	3100
360	2700	2800	3000	3100

	50 year old	Man		
Weight (lbs)	Height (feet)			
	4	5	6	7
110	1100	1200	1400	1500
120	1100	1300	1400	1600
130	1200	1400	1500	1700
140	1300	1400	1600	1700
150	1300	1500	1600	1800
160	1400	1500	1700	1800
170	1400	1600	1800	1900
180	1500	1700	1800	2000
190	1600	1700	1900	2000
200	1600	1800	1900	2100
210	1700	1800	2000	2200
220	1800	1900	2100	2200
230	1800	2000	2100	2300
240	1900	2000	2200	2300
250	1900	2100	2300	2400
260	2000	2200	2300	2500
270	2100	2200	2400	2500
280	2100	2300	2400	2600
290	2200	2300	2500	2700
300	2300	2400	2600	2700
310	2300	2500	2600	2800
320	2400	2500	2700	2800
330	2400	2600	2700	2900
340	2500	2700	2800	3000
350	2600	2700	2900	3000
360	2600	2800	2900	3100

		60 year old	Man	
	Height (feet)			
	4	5	6	7
Weight (lbs)				
110	1000	1200	1300	1500
120	1100	1200	1400	1500
130	1200	1300	1500	1600
140	1200	1400	1500	1700
150	1300	1400	1600	1700
160	1300	1500	1600	1800
170	1400	1600	1700	1900
180	1500	1600	1800	1900
190	1500	1700	1800	2000
200	1600	1700	1900	2000
210	1700	1800	2000	2100
220	1700	1900	2000	2200
230	1800	1900	2100	2200
240	1800	2000	2100	2300
250	1900	2100	2200	2400
260	2000	2100	2300	2400
270	2000	2200	2300	2500
280	2100	2200	2400	2500
290	2100	2300	2500	2600
300	2200	2400	2500	2700
310	2300	2400	2600	2700
320	2300	2500	2600	2800
330	2400	2500	2700	2900
340	2500	2600	2800	2900
350	2500	2700	2800	3000
360	2600	2700	2900	3000

Weight (lbs)	70 year old		Man	
	Height (feet)			
	4	5	6	7
110	1000	1100	1300	1400
120	1000	1200	1300	1500
130	1100	1300	1400	1600
140	1200	1300	1500	1600
150	1200	1400	1500	1700
160	1300	1400	1600	1700
170	1400	1500	1700	1800
180	1400	1600	1700	1900
190	1500	1600	1800	1900
200	1500	1700	1800	2000
210	1600	1800	1900	2100
220	1700	1800	2000	2100
230	1700	1900	2000	2200
240	1800	1900	2100	2200
250	1900	2000	2200	2300
260	1900	2100	2200	2400
270	2000	2100	2300	2400
280	2000	2200	2300	2500
290	2100	2300	2400	2600
300	2200	2300	2500	2600
310	2200	2400	2500	2700
320	2300	2400	2600	2700
330	2400	2500	2700	2800
340	2400	2600	2700	2900
350	2500	2600	2800	2900
360	2500	2700	2800	3000

		80 year old	Man	
		Height (feet)		
	4	5	6	7
Weight (lbs)				
110	900	1100	1200	1400
120	1000	1100	1300	1500
130	1100	1200	1400	1500
140	1100	1300	1400	1600
150	1200	1300	1500	1600
160	1200	1400	1500	1700
170	1300	1500	1600	1800
180	1400	1500	1700	1800
190	1400	1600	1700	1900
200	1500	1600	1800	2000
210	1600	1700	1900	2000
220	1600	1800	1900	2100
230	1700	1800	2000	2100
240	1700	1900	2000	2200
250	1800	2000	2100	2300
260	1900	2000	2200	2300
270	1900	2100	2200	2400
280	2000	2100	2300	2400
290	2100	2200	2400	2500
300	2100	2300	2400	2600
310	2200	2300	2500	2600
320	2200	2400	2500	2700
330	2300	2500	2600	2800
340	2400	2500	2700	2800
350	2400	2600	2700	2900
360	2500	2600	2800	2900

| | 20 year old | Woman | | |
| Height (feet) | | | | |
Weight (lbs)	4	5	6	7
110	1200	1300	1300	1400
120	1300	1300	1400	1400
130	1300	1400	1400	1500
140	1300	1400	1500	1500
150	1400	1400	1500	1600
160	1400	1500	1500	1600
170	1500	1500	1600	1600
180	1500	1600	1600	1700
190	1600	1600	1700	1700
200	1600	1700	1700	1800
210	1700	1700	1800	1800
220	1700	1800	1800	1900
230	1700	1800	1800	1900
240	1800	1800	1900	1900
250	1800	1900	1900	2000
260	1900	1900	2000	2000
270	1900	2000	2000	2100
280	2000	2000	2100	2100
290	2000	2100	2100	2200
300	2000	2100	2200	2200
310	2100	2100	2200	2300
320	2100	2200	2200	2300
330	2200	2200	2300	2300
340	2200	2300	2300	2400
350	2300	2300	2400	2400
360	2300	2400	2400	2500

Weight (lbs)	30 year old Woman Height (feet)			
	4	5	6	7
110	1200	1200	1300	1300
120	1200	1300	1300	1400
130	1300	1300	1400	1400
140	1300	1400	1400	1500
150	1300	1400	1500	1500
160	1400	1400	1500	1600
170	1400	1500	1500	1600
180	1500	1500	1600	1600
190	1500	1600	1600	1700
200	1600	1600	1700	1700
210	1600	1700	1700	1800
220	1600	1700	1800	1800
230	1700	1700	1800	1900
240	1700	1800	1800	1900
250	1800	1800	1900	1900
260	1800	1900	1900	2000
270	1900	1900	2000	2000
280	1900	2000	2000	2100
290	2000	2000	2100	2100
300	2000	2100	2100	2200
310	2000	2100	2200	2200
320	2100	2100	2200	2300
330	2100	2200	2200	2300
340	2200	2200	2300	2300
350	2200	2300	2300	2400
360	2300	2300	2400	2400

	40 year old	Woman		
	Height (feet)			
	4	5	6	7
Weight (lbs)				
110	1100	1200	1200	1300
120	1200	1200	1300	1300
130	1200	1300	1300	1400
140	1300	1300	1400	1400
150	1300	1400	1400	1500
160	1300	1400	1500	1500
170	1400	1400	1500	1600
180	1400	1500	1500	1600
190	1500	1500	1600	1600
200	1500	1600	1600	1700
210	1600	1600	1700	1700
220	1600	1700	1700	1800
230	1600	1700	1800	1800
240	1700	1700	1800	1900
250	1700	1800	1800	1900
260	1800	1800	1900	1900
270	1800	1900	1900	2000
280	1900	1900	2000	2000
290	1900	2000	2000	2100
300	1900	2000	2100	2100
310	2000	2000	2100	2200
320	2000	2100	2100	2200
330	2100	2100	2200	2200
340	2100	2200	2200	2300
350	2200	2200	2300	2300
360	2200	2300	2300	2400

		50 year old	Woman	
	Height (feet)			
	4	5	6	7
Weight (lbs)				
110	1100	1100	1200	1200
120	1100	1200	1200	1300
130	1200	1200	1300	1300
140	1200	1300	1300	1400
150	1200	1300	1400	1400
160	1300	1300	1400	1500
170	1300	1400	1400	1500
180	1400	1400	1500	1500
190	1400	1500	1500	1600
200	1500	1500	1600	1600
210	1500	1600	1600	1700
220	1600	1600	1700	1700
230	1600	1700	1700	1800
240	1600	1700	1800	1800
250	1700	1700	1800	1900
260	1700	1800	1800	1900
270	1800	1800	1900	1900
280	1800	1900	1900	2000
290	1900	1900	2000	2000
300	1900	2000	2000	2100
310	1900	2000	2100	2100
320	2000	2000	2100	2200
330	2000	2100	2100	2200
340	2100	2100	2200	2200
350	2100	2200	2200	2300
360	2200	2200	2300	2300

Weight (lbs)	Height (feet)			
	4	5	6	7
110	1000	1100	1100	1200
120	1100	1100	1200	1200
130	1100	1200	1200	1300
140	1200	1200	1300	1300
150	1200	1300	1300	1400
160	1200	1300	1400	1400
170	1300	1300	1400	1500
180	1300	1400	1400	1500
190	1400	1400	1500	1500
200	1400	1500	1500	1600
210	1500	1500	1600	1600
220	1500	1600	1600	1700
230	1500	1600	1700	1700
240	1600	1600	1700	1800
250	1600	1700	1700	1800
260	1700	1700	1800	1800
270	1700	1800	1800	1900
280	1800	1800	1900	1900
290	1800	1900	1900	2000
300	1900	1900	2000	2000
310	1900	2000	2000	2100
320	1900	2000	2100	2100
330	2000	2000	2100	2200
340	2000	2100	2100	2200
350	2100	2100	2200	2200
360	2100	2200	2200	2300

Weight (lbs)		70 year old		Woman	
		Height (feet)			
	4	5	6	7
110	1000	1000	1100	1100
120	1000	1100	1100	1200
130	1100	1100	1200	1200
140	1100	1200	1200	1300
150	1200	1200	1300	1300
160	1200	1300	1300	1400
170	1200	1300	1400	1400
180	1300	1300	1400	1500
190	1300	1400	1400	1500
200	1400	1400	1500	1500
210	1400	1500	1500	1600
220	1500	1500	1600	1600
230	1500	1600	1600	1700
240	1500	1600	1700	1700
250	1600	1600	1700	1800
260	1600	1700	1700	1800
270	1700	1700	1800	1800
280	1700	1800	1800	1900
290	1800	1800	1900	1900
300	1800	1900	1900	2000
310	1900	1900	2000	2000
320	1900	2000	2000	2100
330	1900	2000	2000	2100
340	2000	2000	2100	2100
350	2000	2100	2100	2200
360	2100	2100	2200	2200

80 year old   Woman

Height (feet)

Weight (lbs)	4	5	6	7
110	900	1000	1000	1100
120	1000	1000	1100	1100
130	1000	1100	1100	1200
140	1100	1100	1200	1200
150	1100	1200	1200	1300
160	1200	1200	1300	1300
170	1200	1300	1300	1400
180	1200	1300	1400	1400
190	1300	1300	1400	1500
200	1300	1400	1400	1500
210	1400	1400	1500	1500
220	1400	1500	1500	1600
230	1500	1500	1600	1600
240	1500	1600	1600	1700
250	1500	1600	1700	1700
260	1600	1600	1700	1800
270	1600	1700	1700	1800
280	1700	1700	1800	1800
290	1700	1800	1800	1900
300	1800	1800	1900	1900
310	1800	1900	1900	2000
320	1800	1900	2000	2000
330	1900	1900	2000	2100
340	1900	2000	2000	2100
350	2000	2000	2100	2100
360	2000	2100	2100	2200

www.ingramcontent.com/pod-product-compliance
Lightning Source LLC
Chambersburg PA
CBHW070045260726
48658CB00002B/741